Orthodontics Health Guide for Beginners

Understanding the Importance of Orthodontics Health

By

Daley Edwin
Copyright@2023

Table of Contents

CHAPTER 1

Introduction

Orthodontics is a specialized branch of dentistry that focuses on diagnosing, preventing, and treating malocclusions, or issues related to the alignment and positioning of teeth and jaws. It plays a vital role in enhancing oral health, facial aesthetics, and overall well-being.

1.1 What is Orthodontics

Orthodontics is the field of dentistry dedicated to correcting misaligned teeth and jaws. The term "orthodontics" is derived from two Greek words: "ortho," meaning straight, and "odontos," meaning tooth. Essentially, it is the science and art of straightening teeth to create a harmonious and functional bite.

At its core, orthodontics is concerned with the alignment and positioning of teeth within the dental arches and the relationship between the upper and lower jaws. It addresses a wide range of dental issues, including overcrowded or widely spaced teeth, overbites, underbites, crossbites, and other irregularities that affect the way teeth and jaws function.

Orthodontic treatment involves the use of various appliances, most notably braces and clear aligners, to gradually move teeth into their proper positions. Orthodontists, who are dental specialists with advanced training in orthodontics, assess patients' dental and facial structures, develop treatment plans, and oversee the entire process of alignment correction.

Beyond purely cosmetic concerns, orthodontics plays a significant role in improving oral health and overall quality of life. Straightening teeth and aligning jaws can address a host of issues that extend beyond aesthetics. Properly aligned teeth are easier to clean, reducing the risk of gum disease, tooth decay, and bad breath. A well-balanced bite ensures that chewing and speaking are more efficient and comfortable. orthodontic treatment can contribute to enhanced self-esteem and confidence, as a beautiful smile often results in increased social and psychological well-being.

1.2 Importance of Orthodontic Health

The importance of orthodontic health cannot be overstated, as it goes far beyond simply achieving a visually appealing smile. Here are some key reasons why orthodontic health matters:

1. Oral Health: Misaligned teeth can create crevices and overlaps that make thorough oral hygiene challenging. This increases the risk of plaque buildup, tooth decay, and gum disease. Properly aligned teeth are easier to clean and maintain, promoting better oral health and reducing the need for extensive dental work.

2. Functional Benefits: Orthodontic treatment can correct issues such as overbites, underbites, and crossbites, which can lead to discomfort, pain, and difficulties in chewing and speaking. A well-aligned bite improves overall oral function and minimizes the risk of jaw joint problems.

3. Confidence and Self-Esteem: A straight, beautiful smile can have a profound impact on an individual's self-confidence and self-esteem. It can enhance social interactions and contribute to a positive self-image, leading to improved mental well-being.

4. Preventing Long-Term Issues: Untreated orthodontic problems can lead to more severe issues in the future. Misaligned teeth can cause excessive wear and tear, increasing the risk of dental fractures and other complications. Addressing these issues early through orthodontic treatment can prevent more extensive and costly dental work later in life.

5. Overall Well-Being: Orthodontic health isn't just about teeth; it's about improving an individual's overall quality of life. By creating a properly aligned and functional oral environment, orthodontics contributes to better overall health and well-being.

orthodontics is a specialized field of dentistry dedicated to improving the alignment and positioning of teeth and jaws. Its importance extends beyond aesthetics, encompassing oral health, functional benefits, psychological well-being, and overall quality of life. Understanding the fundamentals of orthodontics is the first step toward appreciating the impact it can have on individuals of all ages.

1.3 Who Can Benefit from Orthodontic Treatment

Orthodontic treatment is not limited to a particular age group or demographic; it offers numerous benefits to a wide range of individuals. Here's a breakdown of who can benefit from orthodontic treatment:

1. Children and Adolescents:

- **Early Intervention:** Orthodontic treatment is often initiated during childhood or adolescence when the jaw is still growing. Early intervention can correct bite problems, guide tooth eruption, and prevent more severe issues from developing.

- **Preventing Future Problems:** Identifying and addressing orthodontic issues at a young age can prevent the need for more extensive and invasive treatments in adulthood.

- **Aesthetics and Confidence:** For young individuals, achieving a well-aligned smile can significantly boost self-confidence and contribute to a positive self-image.

2. Adults:

- **Cosmetic Improvement:** Many adults seek orthodontic treatment for cosmetic reasons, desiring a straighter and more attractive smile.

- **Oral Health:** Orthodontic treatment can improve oral health by aligning teeth properly, making them easier to clean and reducing the risk of gum disease and tooth decay.

- **Functional Benefits:** Adults may also benefit from orthodontics by addressing bite problems, which can lead to discomfort and difficulty in chewing and speaking.

- **Preventive Measures:** Some adults may have orthodontic issues that were not addressed during childhood. Correcting these problems can prevent further complications and tooth wear.

- **Age Is Not a Barrier:** Contrary to common misconceptions, there is no age limit for orthodontic treatment. Advances in orthodontic technology, such as clear aligners, have made treatment more discreet and accessible for adults.

3. Seniors:

- **Oral Health:** Even in their senior years, individuals can benefit from orthodontic treatment. Properly aligned teeth are easier to maintain, which is crucial for maintaining oral health in later life.

- **Comfort:** Addressing bite problems can alleviate discomfort associated with misaligned teeth and jaws.

- **Improved Nutrition:** A well-aligned bite can make it easier to eat a balanced diet, ensuring that seniors receive the nutrition they need for good health.

- **Enhanced Quality of Life:** Orthodontic treatment can contribute to an improved overall quality of life, making it easier for seniors to speak, eat, and socialize comfortably.

4. Those with Specific Orthodontic Issues:

- **Individuals with Bite Problems:** Overbites, underbites, crossbites, and other bite problems can cause functional issues and discomfort. Orthodontic treatment can correct these issues.

- **Crowded or Spaced Teeth:** Orthodontics can address crowded or widely spaced teeth, improving both aesthetics and oral health.

- **Jaw Joint Issues:** Temporomandibular joint (TMJ) disorders can be alleviated or prevented through orthodontic treatment.

- **Speech Difficulties:** Some speech problems can be linked to dental misalignment, which orthodontics may help resolve.

virtually anyone with orthodontic issues or a desire for improved oral health and aesthetics can benefit from orthodontic treatment. It is a versatile field of dentistry that offers solutions for individuals of all ages, from children and adolescents to adults and seniors. The key is to consult with an orthodontist to determine the most appropriate treatment plan based on individual needs and goals.

CHAPTER 2

Understanding Your Oral Health

Understanding your oral health is the foundation for maintaining a healthy mouth and a beautiful smile throughout your life.

2.1 Basics of Dental Anatomy

Understanding the basic structure of your teeth and mouth is essential for maintaining good oral health. Here are the key components of dental anatomy:

1. Teeth: The human mouth typically contains 32 teeth, including incisors, canines, premolars, and molars. Each type of tooth has a specific function in biting, tearing, and grinding food.

2. Tooth Enamel: The outermost layer of your teeth is called enamel. It is the hardest substance in the human body and protects the inner layers of the tooth.

3. Dentin: Beneath the enamel is dentin, a sensitive tissue that makes up most of the tooth's structure. It contains tiny tubules that transmit pain signals when exposed.

4. Pulp: The pulp is the innermost part of the tooth, containing blood vessels, nerves, and connective tissue. It nourishes the tooth and senses temperature and pressure.

5. Gum Tissue: Also known as gingiva, gum tissue surrounds the teeth and provides a seal around them. Healthy gums are essential for overall oral health.

6. Periodontal Ligament: This ligament attaches the teeth to the jawbone and helps absorb the forces generated during chewing.

7. Jawbone: The bones of the upper and lower jaws support the teeth and provide the foundation for your facial structure.

2.2 Common Dental Issues

Maintaining good oral health involves recognizing and addressing common dental issues that can affect your teeth and gums. Here are some of the most prevalent dental problems:

1. Tooth Decay (Cavities): Tooth decay occurs when bacteria in the mouth produce acids that erode the enamel. It can lead to cavities, which are small holes in the teeth. Prevention includes regular brushing, flossing, and dental check-ups.

2. Gum Disease: Gum disease, or periodontal disease, is an infection of the gums and supporting structures of the teeth. It ranges from mild gingivitis to severe periodontitis and can result in tooth loss if left untreated. Good oral hygiene is crucial for prevention.

3. Tooth Sensitivity: Sensitivity occurs when the dentin is exposed, leading to discomfort when consuming hot, cold, sweet, or acidic foods or beverages. Desensitizing toothpaste and professional treatments can alleviate sensitivity.

4. Bad Breath (Halitosis): Bad breath can be caused by poor oral hygiene, gum disease, dry mouth, or underlying medical conditions. Regular brushing, flossing, and tongue cleaning can help combat bad breath.

5. Teeth Grinding (Bruxism): Bruxism involves clenching or grinding your teeth, often during sleep. It can lead to tooth damage, headaches, and jaw pain. Mouthguards or lifestyle changes can help manage bruxism.

6. Crooked or Misaligned Teeth: Crooked teeth can affect both aesthetics and oral function. Orthodontic treatment, such as braces or clear aligners, can straighten teeth and improve bite alignment.

7. Tooth Loss: Tooth loss can occur due to decay, gum disease, injury, or other factors. Options for tooth replacement include dental implants, bridges, and dentures.

8. Oral Cancer: Oral cancer can develop in the mouth, throat, or lips. Early detection through regular dental check-ups is crucial for successful treatment.

Understanding the basics of dental anatomy and being aware of common dental issues, you can take proactive steps to maintain your oral health. Regular dental visits, proper oral hygiene practices, and a healthy lifestyle are essential components of a lifelong commitment to a healthy smile.

2.3 How Orthodontics Fits into Oral Health

Orthodontics plays a significant role in enhancing and maintaining oral health by addressing issues related to the alignment and positioning of teeth and jaws. Here's how orthodontics fits into oral health:

1. Correcting Misalignment: One of the primary purposes of orthodontic treatment is to correct misaligned teeth and jaws. When teeth are crooked, overcrowded, or improperly spaced, it can be challenging to clean them effectively, leading to a higher risk of dental problems like tooth decay and gum disease. Orthodontics helps align teeth properly, making them easier to clean and reducing the likelihood of these issues.

2. Improving Bite Function:
Orthodontic treatment can correct bite problems such as overbites, underbites, and crossbites. A well-aligned bite ensures that the upper and lower teeth fit together correctly when chewing and speaking. This not only enhances oral function but also minimizes the risk of jaw joint problems and discomfort associated with improper bite alignment.

3. Enhancing Speech: In some cases, dental misalignment can contribute to speech difficulties. Orthodontic treatment can help improve speech clarity and pronunciation by addressing the underlying alignment issues that may be affecting speech patterns.

4. Preventing Dental Wear and Damage: Teeth that are misaligned or bite improperly can experience excessive wear and damage over time. By aligning teeth and jaws, orthodontics can prevent premature dental erosion and the need for restorative dental procedures.

5. Supporting Overall Health: Poor oral health has been linked to various systemic health issues, including heart disease, diabetes, and respiratory problems. Orthodontic treatment can contribute to better oral health, reducing the risk of these potential health concerns.

6. Enhancing Aesthetics and Self-Esteem: While aesthetics is not the sole focus of orthodontics, they are an essential aspect. A beautifully aligned smile can boost an individual's self-esteem and confidence, leading to improved overall well-being and a more positive self-image.

7. Long-Term Benefits: Orthodontic treatment can provide long-term benefits that extend well beyond the duration of the treatment itself. Maintaining proper alignment and bite function can contribute to a lifetime of oral health and comfort.

orthodontics is a crucial component of oral health care, addressing issues related to tooth and jaw alignment that can impact not only the aesthetics of a smile but also overall oral function and well-being. By ensuring that teeth and jaws are properly aligned, orthodontics plays a vital role in preventing dental problems, improving oral function, and supporting overall health.

CHAPTER 3

Types of Orthodontic Problems

Orthodontic problems encompass a range of issues related to the alignment and positioning of teeth and jaws. Addressing these problems is the primary goal of orthodontic treatment.

3.1 Malocclusion: The Key Issue

Malocclusion is a term used to describe the improper alignment of teeth when the upper and lower dental arches do not fit together correctly. It is often considered the key issue in orthodontics as it underlies many other dental alignment problems. Malocclusion can manifest in various forms, including:

- **Overbite:** An overbite occurs when the upper front teeth overlap significantly with the lower front teeth when the jaws are closed. This can result in the upper teeth biting over the lower teeth, potentially leading to wear and tear on the lower teeth.

- **Underbite:** In contrast, an underbite occurs when the lower front teeth protrude further than the upper front teeth. This can affect speech and bite function and may cause jaw discomfort.

- **Crossbite:** Crossbite refers to a situation where some upper teeth sit inside the lower teeth when biting down, while others are outside. This can lead to uneven wear on teeth and may cause jaw misalignment.

- **Open Bite:** An open bite occurs when the upper and lower front teeth do not meet when the jaws are closed. This can lead to speech problems and difficulty biting into food.

- **Midline Misalignment:** Midline misalignment occurs when the center lines of the upper and lower teeth do not align properly. This can result in an uneven smile.

Malocclusion can vary in severity, and its correction is a primary focus of orthodontic treatment. Treatment options may include braces, clear aligners, headgear, or other orthodontic devices tailored to the specific malocclusion.

3.2 Crowding and Spacing

Crowding and **spacing** are common orthodontic problems related to the arrangement of teeth within the dental arches:

- **Crowding:** Crowding occurs when there is insufficient space within the jaw for all the teeth to align correctly. This can cause teeth to overlap, twist, or become misaligned. Crowding not only affects aesthetics but also makes proper oral hygiene challenging, increasing the risk of tooth decay and gum disease.

- **Spacing:** Spacing issues, on the other hand, involve gaps or spaces between teeth that are larger than normal. While some spacing between teeth is natural and may not pose a problem, excessive spacing can impact bite function and aesthetics. It can also lead to food getting stuck between teeth, increasing the risk of decay.

Both crowding and spacing can be addressed through orthodontic treatment. For crowding, orthodontics can create additional space or align teeth properly. Spacing issues can be addressed by closing gaps using braces or aligners. The goal is to achieve a harmonious and functional alignment of teeth within the dental arches.

3.3 Overbites, Underbites, and Crossbites

Overbites, underbites, and crossbites are common orthodontic issues related to the alignment of the upper and lower teeth and jaws:

Overbite: An **overbite** occurs when the upper front teeth significantly overlap the lower front teeth when the jaws are closed. This condition is also known as "buck teeth." Overbites can lead to aesthetic concerns, but more importantly, they can affect bite function and may cause excessive wear on the lower teeth.

Underbite: In contrast, an **underbite** occurs when the lower front teeth protrude further than the upper front teeth, causing the lower jaw to jut forward. This misalignment can impact speech and bite function and may lead to jaw discomfort and difficulties with oral hygiene.

Crossbite: A **crossbite** refers to a situation where some upper teeth sit inside the lower teeth when biting down, while others are outside. Crossbites can result in uneven wear on teeth, jaw misalignment, and difficulty with proper dental function.

These bite issues can vary in severity, and treatment options may include braces, clear aligners, orthodontic appliances, or even jaw surgery in more extreme cases. Correcting these problems is essential not only for aesthetics but also for overall oral health and function.

3.4 Other Orthodontic Concerns

In addition to malocclusion, crowding, spacing, overbites, underbites, and crossbites, orthodontic concerns encompass a wide range of issues related to tooth and jaw alignment. Here are some other orthodontic concerns:

- **Open Bite:** An **open bite** occurs when the upper and lower front teeth do not meet when the jaws are closed. This can lead to speech difficulties and challenges when biting into food.

- **Dental Midline Misalignment: Midline misalignment** happens when the center lines of the upper and lower teeth do not align correctly, resulting in an uneven smile.

- **Impacted Teeth:** Some teeth may fail to erupt properly, becoming **impacted** or trapped beneath the gumline. Orthodontic treatment may be needed to create space for these teeth to emerge.

- **Supernumerary Teeth:** Occasionally, individuals may have extra teeth, known as **supernumerary teeth**, which can disrupt the natural alignment of the dental arches.

- **Orthodontic Relapse:** Sometimes, orthodontic treatment results may regress over time, requiring follow-up treatment to maintain the alignment achieved during the initial treatment.

- **Orthodontic Retention:** After orthodontic treatment, the use of **retainers** is often necessary to prevent teeth from shifting back to their original positions. Retention is a crucial aspect of long-term treatment success.

Orthodontists are trained to diagnose and address these and many other orthodontic concerns. The choice of treatment depends on the specific issue, its severity, and the individual's unique needs and goals. Orthodontic care aims to create a functional and aesthetically pleasing alignment of teeth and jaws while promoting long-term oral health and well-being.

CHAPTER 4

Orthodontic Treatment Options

Orthodontic treatment has evolved significantly over the years, offering various options to address issues related to tooth and jaw alignment.

4.1 Braces: Traditional and Modern Types

Traditional Braces: Traditional braces are a well-established and effective orthodontic treatment option. They consist of several key components:

- **Brackets:** Brackets are small metal or ceramic attachments bonded to the front surfaces of the teeth. These brackets serve as anchor points for other parts of the braces.

- **Archwires:** Archwires are thin, flexible wires that run through the brackets and are attached to them using tiny bands called ligatures. The archwire applies gentle pressure to move the teeth into their desired positions.

- **Bands:** Bands are metal rings that encircle the molars or anchor teeth and are connected to the archwire. They provide stability and support for the entire system.

- **Elastics:** Elastics, also known as rubber bands, are sometimes used to correct bite problems or to move specific teeth into proper alignment.

Traditional braces are highly effective for treating a wide range of orthodontic issues, including severe misalignments and complex cases. They are particularly useful for cases where significant tooth movement is required.

Modern Types of Braces:
Advancements in orthodontics have led to several modern types of braces that offer more discreet and comfortable options:

- **Ceramic Braces:** Ceramic braces use tooth-colored or clear brackets, making them less noticeable than traditional metal braces. They are a popular choice among individuals who desire a more aesthetic treatment option.

- **Lingual Braces:** Lingual braces are attached to the back (lingual) surfaces of the teeth, making them virtually invisible from the front. They are an excellent choice for those who want a discreet treatment option.

- **Self-Ligating Braces:** Self-ligating braces use special brackets that do not require ligatures (bands) to hold the archwire in place. They are known for reduced friction and shorter treatment times.

4.2 Clear Aligners

Clear aligners represent a modern and increasingly popular orthodontic treatment option. They are a series of custom-made, clear plastic trays that fit snugly over the teeth. Clear aligners, such as those provided by Invisalign, have several advantages:

- **Aesthetic Appeal:** Clear aligners are nearly invisible, making them a discreet choice for individuals who prefer a less noticeable treatment option.

- **Removability:** Aligners can be easily removed for eating, drinking, brushing, and flossing, allowing for better oral hygiene and dietary flexibility during treatment.

- **Comfort:** Aligners are smooth and comfortable to wear, with no sharp edges or wires to cause irritation to the cheeks and lips.

- **Predictable Treatment:** Advanced computer technology is used to plan and predict the movements of teeth, ensuring efficient and precise treatment.

Clear aligners are effective for addressing mild to moderate orthodontic issues, including crowding, spacing, and minor bite problems. They are not suitable for all cases, especially those requiring significant tooth or jaw movement.

The choice between traditional braces and clear aligners depends on individual needs, treatment goals, and the recommendation of the orthodontist. Both options offer effective solutions for achieving a well-aligned and healthy smile, and the decision should be based on a thorough evaluation and discussion with a qualified orthodontic specialist.

4.3 Other Orthodontic Devices

Orthodontics encompasses a variety of devices beyond traditional braces and clear aligners to address specific orthodontic issues. These devices serve as valuable tools in the hands of orthodontists to achieve optimal results:

- **Headgear:** Headgear is a device that consists of a strap worn around the head or neck and wires attached to the braces. It is primarily used to correct severe bite problems by exerting external force on the upper or lower jaw.

- **Palatal Expanders:** Palatal expanders are used to widen the upper jaw when it is too narrow to accommodate all of the permanent teeth. They are particularly useful for children with crowding issues.

- **Retainers:** Retainers are appliances worn after active orthodontic treatment to maintain the results. They prevent teeth from shifting back to their original positions. There are both removable and fixed (bonded) retainers.

- **Functional Appliances:** Functional appliances are often used in younger patients to correct bite issues by modifying jaw growth and positioning.

- **Space Maintainers:** Space maintainers are used in children to preserve the space left by a prematurely lost baby tooth, preventing adjacent teeth from shifting and maintaining proper alignment.

4.4 Pros and Cons of Different Treatments

Each orthodontic treatment option comes with its own set of advantages and disadvantages, which should be considered when making a decision:

Pros of Braces (Traditional and Modern Types):

- Effective for a wide range of orthodontic issues, including complex cases.

- Controlled and predictable tooth movement.

- May be more suitable for severe misalignments.

- No compliance concerns since they are fixed in place.

- Modern options offer aesthetics and comfort improvements.

Cons of Braces:

- Visible metal or ceramic brackets and wires.

- Dietary restrictions due to the risk of damage to braces.

- Slightly more challenging oral hygiene compared to clear aligners.

- Potential for discomfort and occasional adjustments.

Pros of Clear Aligners:

- Virtually invisible, offering aesthetic advantages.

- Removable for eating, brushing, and flossing.

- Smooth and comfortable to wear.

- No dietary restrictions.

- Fewer office visits for adjustments.

Cons of Clear Aligners:

- Not suitable for severe orthodontic problems.

- Require diligent compliance to achieve desired results.

- May cause initial speech challenges.

- Higher cost compared to traditional braces in some cases.

- Potential for loss or damage if not handled properly.

Pros of Other Orthodontic Devices:

- Targeted solutions for specific issues.

- Can be highly effective for complex cases.

- May reduce the need for more invasive treatments like jaw surgery.

- Can facilitate early intervention in children, preventing severe problems later.

Cons of Other Orthodontic Devices:

- Often require more active patient compliance.

- Some devices, like headgear, may be less comfortable and less discreet.

- May involve longer treatment times for comprehensive results.

- Require regular adjustments and monitoring by the orthodontist.

The choice of orthodontic treatment should be made in consultation with an orthodontic specialist who can evaluate individual needs, preferences, and the specific nature of the orthodontic issues. Ultimately, the goal is to select the treatment that will provide the best outcome in terms of alignment, oral health, and patient satisfaction.

CHAPTER 5

The Orthodontic Journey

The orthodontic journey is a structured process that guides individuals through the steps of diagnosis, treatment planning, and the actual orthodontic treatment with the goal of achieving a healthy and well-aligned smile. Here's an overview of the key stages in this journey:

5.1 The Initial Consultation

The initial consultation is the first step in the orthodontic journey and serves as the foundation for the entire process. During this crucial appointment:

- **Assessment:** The orthodontist will conduct a comprehensive evaluation of your oral health, which may include taking X-rays, photographs, and impressions of your teeth. They will assess your dental and facial structure, bite alignment, and any existing orthodontic issues.

- **Medical and Dental History:** You will provide information about your medical and dental history, including any previous dental treatments or surgeries, allergies, medications, and habits like thumb-sucking or nail-biting.

- **Discussion of Concerns:** This is an opportunity to discuss any concerns you have about your teeth, jaw, or smile. Be sure to mention any discomfort, pain, or aesthetic preferences.

- **Treatment Options:** The orthodontist will explain the orthodontic treatment options suitable for your specific needs and discuss their recommendations. This may include traditional braces, clear aligners, or other devices.

- **Cost and Timeline:** You will receive an estimate of the treatment duration and cost. The orthodontic team will also provide information about insurance coverage and payment plans.

- **Questions and Clarifications:** It's essential to ask any questions and seek clarifications about the proposed treatment plan, expected outcomes, and potential alternatives.

5.2 Treatment Planning

After the initial consultation, the orthodontist will proceed with treatment planning. This involves:

- **Diagnostic Analysis:** Reviewing the collected data, such as X-rays and impressions, to create a precise diagnosis of your orthodontic issues.

- **Customized Treatment Plan:** Based on the diagnosis, the orthodontist will develop a personalized treatment plan tailored to your needs and goals. This plan outlines the steps necessary to achieve the desired results.

- **Device Selection:** Determining which orthodontic device or technique is best suited to address your specific concerns. This decision may take into account factors like aesthetics, comfort, and treatment duration.

- **Treatment Phases:** Breaking down the treatment into phases, if necessary, and outlining the expected progress at each stage. For example, a multi-phase plan may involve addressing bite issues before straightening teeth.

- **Monitoring and Adjustments:** Establishing a schedule for regular check-ups and adjustments throughout the treatment to ensure that your progress aligns with the treatment plan.

5.3 Getting Braces or Aligners

Once the treatment plan is finalized, the next step is to start the orthodontic treatment, which typically involves getting braces or aligners:

- **Braces:** If you opt for traditional braces, the orthodontist will begin by attaching brackets to your teeth using a dental adhesive. Archwires and ligatures will be placed to connect the brackets and guide tooth movement. You may experience some discomfort initially, and regular adjustments will be necessary to tighten the braces.

- **Aligners:** If you choose clear aligners, a series of custom-made trays will be created to fit over your teeth. You'll wear each set of aligners for a specified period, typically two weeks, before moving on to the next set. Aligners should be worn for most of the day and night, except when eating or cleaning your teeth.

- **Oral Hygiene and Care:** Regardless of the treatment option, maintaining excellent oral hygiene is crucial. You will receive guidance on how to clean your teeth, braces, or aligners effectively and avoid foods that could damage your orthodontic devices.

- **Regular Check-ups:** You'll attend regular appointments with your orthodontist for adjustments, progress monitoring, and to address any issues or concerns that may arise during treatment.

The orthodontic journey can vary in duration depending on individual needs and the complexity of the treatment plan. However, it ultimately leads to a beautifully aligned smile and improved oral health. Communication with your orthodontist and adherence to their recommendations are key factors in a successful orthodontic journey.

5.4 Maintenance and Regular Checkups

Maintenance and regular checkups are essential components of any orthodontic treatment journey. These ongoing aspects of orthodontic care are crucial for ensuring that your teeth remain properly aligned and that your treatment progresses as planned. Here's what you need to know about maintenance and regular checkups during orthodontic treatment:

Maintenance and Oral Hygiene:

1. **Oral Hygiene:** Proper oral hygiene is vital throughout your orthodontic treatment. Maintaining a clean and healthy mouth helps prevent issues like tooth decay and gum disease. Brush your teeth thoroughly, including around brackets or aligners, and use floss or interdental brushes to clean between teeth and wires.

2. **Dietary Considerations:** Continue to be mindful of your diet. Avoid hard, sticky, and overly sugary foods that can damage braces or aligners. It's best to stick to a balanced and tooth-friendly diet.

3. **Orthodontic Device Care:** If you have braces, be careful not to damage the brackets or wires when eating. If you wear clear aligners, clean them as instructed by your orthodontist to prevent bacteria buildup.

Regular Checkups:

1. **Appointment Schedule:** Your orthodontist will schedule regular check-up appointments throughout your treatment. These appointments are crucial for monitoring your progress and making any necessary adjustments.

2. **Adjustments:** During these appointments, your orthodontist may adjust your braces or provide you with a new set of aligners. These adjustments are

essential to ensure that your teeth continue to move toward their desired positions.

3. **Progress Assessment:** Your orthodontist will evaluate how well your teeth are responding to treatment and whether any modifications to the treatment plan are necessary. They may also assess your bite alignment and overall oral health.

4. **Addressing Concerns:** If you experience any discomfort or have concerns about your treatment between scheduled appointments, don't hesitate to contact your orthodontist. They can provide guidance and address any issues promptly.

5. **Retention:** Toward the end of your active orthodontic

treatment, your orthodontist will discuss the transition to the retention phase. This phase typically involves the use of retainers to maintain the alignment achieved during treatment.

Retention Phase:

1. **Retainers:** Retainers are custom-made devices that help keep your teeth in their newly aligned positions. They may be removable or fixed (bonded) behind your teeth.

2. **Compliance:** Following your orthodontist's instructions for retainer wear is essential to prevent your teeth from shifting back to their original positions. Initially, you may need to wear your retainers all the time,

gradually transitioning to nighttime wear.

3. **Regular Retainer Checkups:** Even during the retention phase, it's essential to attend regular check-up appointments with your orthodontist. They will monitor your retention progress and make any necessary adjustments.

Maintenance and regular checkups are integral to the long-term success of your orthodontic treatment. By following your orthodontist's recommendations, maintaining excellent oral hygiene, attending scheduled appointments, and wearing retainers as instructed, you can enjoy a beautiful, healthy smile that lasts a lifetime.

CHAPTER 6

Caring for Your Orthodontic Appliances

Caring for your orthodontic appliances, whether you have braces or clear aligners, is crucial to ensure the success of your treatment and maintain good oral health. Here are guidelines for caring for orthodontic appliances:

6.1 Proper Oral Hygiene with Braces

Braces require careful attention to oral hygiene to prevent issues like tooth decay and gum disease. Here's how to maintain proper oral hygiene with braces:

- **Regular Brushing:** Brush your teeth after every meal and before bedtime using a soft-bristle toothbrush. Angle the brush toward the brackets and gums to clean around them. Pay special attention to the areas where the brackets and wires meet your teeth.

- **Interdental Brushes:** Use interdental brushes or proxy brushes to clean between wires and brackets. These small brushes can reach areas that regular brushing may miss.

- **Flossing:** Flossing can be more challenging with braces, but it's essential. Use floss threaders or orthodontic floss to pass under the archwire and between teeth. Consider using a water flosser for added convenience.

- **Fluoride Mouthwash:** Rinse with a fluoride mouthwash daily to help strengthen your teeth and prevent tooth decay. Swish it around your mouth for about 30 seconds and then spit it out.

- **Regular Checkups:** Maintain your regular dental checkup appointments. Your orthodontist and dentist will work together to ensure your oral health is on track during orthodontic treatment.

- **Avoid Problematic Foods:** Steer clear of hard, sticky, and overly sugary foods that can damage brackets and wires. Foods like popcorn, gum, caramel, and hard candies should be avoided.

- **Orthodontic Wax:** Use orthodontic wax if you experience any irritation or sore spots from brackets or wires. Apply a small amount to the problem area to provide relief.

6.2 Cleaning Clear Aligners

Clear aligners offer a different set of care instructions compared to braces. Here's how to properly clean and maintain clear aligners:

- **Remove Before Eating or Drinking:** Always remove your clear aligners before eating or drinking anything other than water. Eating or drinking with aligners in place can damage them and increase the risk of staining.

- **Rinse After Removal:** After removing your aligners, rinse them with lukewarm water to remove saliva and food particles. Avoid using hot water, as it can deform the aligners.

- **Brush Your Teeth:** Brush your teeth thoroughly after eating or drinking before putting your aligners back in. This helps prevent staining and the buildup of bacteria.

- **Clean Aligners:** Use a soft toothbrush to gently clean your aligners. Avoid using toothpaste, as it can scratch the aligner material. You can use clear, mild soap or specialized aligner cleaning crystals.

- **Soak in a Cleaning Solution:** Some aligner cleaning solutions are available, or you can create a solution by mixing equal parts water and hydrogen peroxide. Soak your aligners in this solution for 15-20 minutes daily to help maintain their clarity and cleanliness.

- **Store Properly:** When not wearing your aligners, store them in their designated case to prevent loss or damage.

- **Follow the Schedule:** Adhere to your orthodontist's prescribed aligner wear schedule. Consistency is essential for achieving the desired results.

Following these guidelines for proper oral hygiene with braces or clear aligners, you can maintain your appliances effectively, prevent oral health issues, and ensure a successful orthodontic treatment outcome. If you have any questions or concerns about caring for your orthodontic appliances, don't hesitate to consult with your orthodontist.

6.3 Dealing with Discomfort

Orthodontic treatment, whether with braces or clear aligners, may occasionally cause discomfort or soreness. This discomfort is typically temporary and can be managed with some simple strategies. Here's how to deal with discomfort during orthodontic treatment:

1. Saltwater Rinse:

- Dissolve half a teaspoon of salt in eight ounces of warm water.

- Swish the saltwater solution gently in your mouth for about 30 seconds, then spit it out.

- This can help reduce inflammation and ease discomfort.

2. Over-the-Counter Pain Relievers:

- Non-prescription pain relievers such as ibuprofen (Advil) or acetaminophen (Tylenol) can help alleviate pain.

- Follow the recommended dosage instructions on the packaging and consult with your orthodontist or dentist if you have any concerns.

3. Orthodontic Wax:

- If brackets or wires are causing irritation or sore spots inside your mouth, you can apply orthodontic wax to those areas.

- Roll a small piece of wax into a ball and place it over the sharp or irritating spot. The wax creates a smooth barrier.

4. Cold Compress:

- If you experience jaw discomfort or swelling, you can apply a cold compress to the outside of your face.

- Use a clean cloth or ice pack wrapped in a towel and apply it for 15-20 minutes at a time with breaks in between.

5. Soft Diet:

- Stick to a soft diet if you have pain or soreness, especially right after an adjustment.

- Foods like yogurt, mashed potatoes, soup, and smoothies can be more comfortable to eat.

6. Follow Orthodontic Instructions:

- Ensure that you are following your orthodontist's instructions regarding the use of elastics, headgear, or other orthodontic devices.

- Proper use of these devices can help reduce discomfort and achieve the desired results more efficiently.

7. Keep Your Mouth Clean:

- Maintaining excellent oral hygiene is crucial during orthodontic treatment.

- Clean your teeth, braces, or aligners thoroughly to prevent additional discomfort from issues like food particles getting stuck.

8. Communicate with Your Orthodontist:

- If you experience persistent or severe discomfort, contact your orthodontist's office. They can provide guidance and may be able to adjust your appliances or treatment plan to reduce discomfort.

9. Patience:

- Remember that some discomfort is normal during orthodontic treatment as your teeth are gradually moving. It typically improves within a few days to a week after adjustments.

It's important to keep in mind that discomfort is a natural part of the orthodontic process as your teeth adjust to their new positions. However, if you ever experience severe pain, broken appliances, or other issues that require immediate attention, contact your orthodontist as soon as possible. They are there to help you throughout your orthodontic journey and can provide solutions to make your treatment as comfortable as possible.

CHAPTER 7

Dietary Guidelines during Orthodontic Treatment

Maintaining a proper diet is crucial during orthodontic treatment to protect your braces or aligners and promote oral health. Here are some dietary guidelines to follow, starting with foods to avoid:

7.1 Foods to Avoid

1. **Hard Foods:** Hard foods can damage braces, brackets, and wires. Avoid items like:

- Nuts and seeds

- Hard candies

- Ice cubes or ice chips

- Popcorn (especially unpopped kernels)

- Hard pretzels

- Crunchy granola bars

2. **Sticky and Chewy Foods:** Sticky or chewy foods can get stuck in braces and are challenging to clean. They include:

- Caramels

- Taffy

- Chewy candies

- Gum (even sugar-free gum)

3. **Crunchy Fruits and Vegetables:** Some hard fruits and vegetables

can be difficult to bite into. Instead, cook or cut them into small, manageable pieces. Examples include:

- Apples (sliced)

- Carrots (cooked or thinly sliced)

- Raw celery

4. **Tough Meats:** Meats that are tough to chew can be challenging with braces. Consider cutting meat into smaller portions and removing bones. Tough meats include:

- Steak (cut into small pieces)

- Ribs (meat removed from the bone)

- Jerky

5. **Bread with Hard Crusts:** Be cautious with bread that has hard

crusts, like baguettes or certain artisan bread. Soften crusts or opt for softer bread varieties.

6. **Corn on the Cob:** Corn on the cob can be problematic with braces. Consider removing the corn from the cob before eating.

7. **Whole Fruits:** Whole fruits like apples and pears can be challenging to bite into. It's best to slice them into smaller pieces to avoid strain on your braces.

8. **Sugary and Acidic Foods:** Excessive sugar and acid can lead to tooth decay and erosion. Limit the consumption of sugary snacks and acidic beverages. If you indulge in sweets or acidic drinks, make sure to brush your teeth afterward.

9. **Biting with Front Teeth:** Avoid biting directly into hard foods with your front teeth, as this can damage brackets and wires. Use your back teeth for chewing.

10. **Food with Excessive Color:** Some foods and beverages can stain clear aligners. Try to minimize the consumption of foods like curry, berries, and dark-colored sauces.

These guidelines are intended to protect your orthodontic appliances and maintain good oral hygiene. Adhering to them will help ensure that your treatment progresses smoothly and that you minimize the risk of damage or complications. Your orthodontist can provide specific dietary advice tailored to your treatment plan.

7.2 Foods that are Braces-Friendly

While some foods should be avoided during orthodontic treatment, there are plenty of braces-friendly options that are less likely to cause damage or discomfort. Here are foods that are generally safe to consume with braces:

1. **Soft Fruits:** opt for softer fruits that can be easily sliced into bite-sized pieces, such as bananas, berries, melons, and grapes.

2. **Cooked Vegetables:** Cooked vegetables are generally easier to chew and gentler on braces. Consider steamed or roasted

options like broccoli, carrots, and cauliflower.

3. **Dairy Products:** Dairy products like yogurt, milk, and cheese are great sources of calcium and protein and are easy on braces.

4. **Soft Breads:** Choose softer bread varieties, like sandwich bread, pitas, and tortillas, which are less likely to damage braces.

5. **Lean Meats:** Select lean cuts of meat that are easy to chew, such as chicken, turkey, and tender cuts of beef. It's a good practice to cut meat into smaller pieces.

6. **Pasta and Rice:** Soft pasta and rice dishes, like macaroni and cheese or risotto, are braces-friendly options.

7. **Soft Snacks:** opt for snacks that are easy to chew, such as pudding, smoothies, soft cookies, and crackers.

8. **Eggs:** Eggs can be prepared in various ways, such as scrambled, boiled, or as omelets, and are braces-friendly sources of protein.

9. **Seafood:** Soft, flaky fish like salmon or tilapia are easy to chew and a healthy choice.

10. **Soup:** Many soups, especially those with softer ingredients, can be enjoyed with braces.

7.3 Maintaining a Balanced Diet

While following braces-friendly food choices, it's essential to maintain a balanced diet that provides all the necessary nutrients for overall health and well-being. Here are tips for maintaining a balanced diet during orthodontic treatment:

1. **Fruits and Vegetables:** Include a variety of fruits and vegetables in your diet to get essential vitamins and fiber. Cooked or sliced options are often easier to manage with braces.

2. **Protein:** Incorporate lean protein sources such as poultry, fish, lean meats, beans, and tofu into your meals for muscle and tissue repair.

3. **Dairy:** Consume dairy products like yogurt, cheese, and milk for calcium, which is crucial for strong teeth and bones.

4. **Whole Grains:** Choose whole grain options like whole wheat

bread, brown rice, and whole grain pasta for fiber and sustained energy.

5. **Limit Sugary and Acidic Foods:** Minimize sugary snacks, soft drinks, and acidic foods to protect your teeth from decay and erosion. If you indulge, brush your teeth afterward.

6. **Hydration:** Drink plenty of water throughout the day to stay hydrated and maintain overall health.

7. **Moderation:** While some treats should be enjoyed in moderation, aim for a balanced diet overall. Avoid excessive consumption of sugary or processed foods.

8. **Consult with a Dietitian:** If you have specific dietary concerns or restrictions, consider consulting

with a registered dietitian who can help you plan a balanced diet tailored to your needs.

Maintaining a balanced diet not only supports your orthodontic treatment but also contributes to your overall health and well-being. By making smart food choices and caring for your braces or aligners, you can ensure a successful orthodontic journey and a healthy smile.

CHAPTER 8

Orthodontics and Lifestyle

Orthodontic treatment can impact various aspects of your lifestyle, including sports, speech, and social and psychological aspects. Here, we'll explore each of these areas:

8.1 Orthodontics and Sports

Participating in sports and physical activities is essential for maintaining a healthy lifestyle. If you're involved in sports while undergoing orthodontic treatment, here are some considerations:

- **Mouthguards:** If you play contact sports or engage in activities with a risk of facial injury, it's essential to wear a mouthguard. Your orthodontist can provide custom-fitted mouthguards that offer the best protection for your teeth and orthodontic appliances.

- **Braces-Friendly Sports:** Some sports pose a lower risk of orthodontic injury. Consider participating in non-contact or low-contact sports during your treatment to minimize the risk of damage to your braces or aligners.

- **Communication:** Communicate with your orthodontist about your sports activities and any concerns you have. They can offer guidance on protecting your orthodontic appliances while staying active.

- **Emergency Plan:** Be prepared for orthodontic emergencies, such as a loose bracket or wire, while participating in sports. Carry orthodontic wax and know how to address minor issues until you can see your orthodontist.

8.2 Orthodontics and Speech

Orthodontic treatment can temporarily affect speech for some individuals.

Here's how it can impact speech and tips for managing these changes:

- **Initial Adjustment:** When braces or aligners are first placed, you may notice changes in your speech as your tongue and lips adapt to the new appliances. This is temporary and typically resolves within a few days to a week.

- **Speech Exercises:** If speech challenges persist, consider practicing speech exercises recommended by your orthodontist or speech therapist to help you adjust to the appliances.

- **Lisp:** Some individuals may experience a temporary lisp when pronouncing certain sounds due to braces or aligners. Regular practice and patience can help overcome this issue.

- **Consult Your Orthodontist:** If speech issues persist or worsen, consult your orthodontist. They can make adjustments or provide guidance to address the problem.

8.3 Social and Psychological Aspects

Orthodontic treatment can have social and psychological implications, especially for adolescents and adults. Here are some considerations:

- **Aesthetic Concerns:** Braces or aligners may impact your self-confidence temporarily due to their appearance. However, remember that they are a means to achieving a more confident and beautiful smile in the long run.

- **Communication:** Discuss your orthodontic treatment with friends and family to keep them informed. They can provide support and encouragement during your orthodontic journey.

- **Educate Yourself:** Learn about the benefits of orthodontic treatment and focus on the positive aspects, such as improved oral health, enhanced aesthetics, and increased self-esteem.

- **Support Groups:** Consider joining orthodontic support groups or online communities to connect with others going through similar experiences. Sharing experiences and tips can be helpful.

- **Personal Growth:** Orthodontic treatment can be a period of personal growth, resilience, and patience. Embrace the journey as an opportunity for self-improvement.

- **Visualize the End Result:** Keep in mind the end result of your orthodontic treatment—a beautifully aligned smile. Visualizing your future smile can provide motivation and excitement.

- **Open Communication:** If you're feeling anxious or overwhelmed about your treatment, don't hesitate to communicate with your orthodontist. They can address your concerns and provide guidance to make the process more comfortable.

Orthodontic treatment is a temporary phase that can lead to long-term benefits in terms of oral health and self-confidence. Embrace the positive aspects of your orthodontic journey and seek support and guidance when needed to make the process smoother and more enjoyable.

CHAPTER 9

After Orthodontic Treatment

Completing orthodontic treatment is a significant achievement, but it's not the end of your journey to maintain a beautiful, healthy smile. Here are key aspects of post-orthodontic treatment care:

9.1 Retainers: Why They're Important

Retainers are an integral part of post-orthodontic treatment care. Here's why they're crucial:

- **Retention:** After your braces or clear aligners are removed, your teeth may have a tendency to shift back to their original positions. Retainers help maintain the new alignment achieved during treatment.

- **Stabilization:** Retainers allow the bone and surrounding tissues to adapt to the new positions of your teeth, ensuring long-term stability.

- **Custom Fit:** Retainers are custom-made to fit your teeth precisely, making them highly effective in preserving your smile's alignment.

- **Types of Retainers:** There are two main types of retainers— removable and fixed (bonded) retainers. Your orthodontist will recommend the type that suits your specific needs.

- **Adjustments:** Over time, your orthodontist may make adjustments to your retainers to ensure they continue to fit properly and effectively.

- **Compliance:** It's crucial to follow your orthodontist's instructions regarding retainer wear. Initially, you may need to wear them full-time and gradually transition to nighttime wear.

- **Long-Term Use:** In many cases, retainers are worn indefinitely, with nighttime wear being the long-term maintenance phase.

Consistency in wearing them is essential for preserving your smile.

9.2 Post-Treatment Oral Care

Maintaining excellent oral care practices is essential for long-term oral health and the preservation of your new smile:

- **Regular Dental Checkups:** Continue seeing your dentist for regular checkups and cleanings, typically every six months. These visits help monitor your oral health and address any issues promptly.

- **Orthodontic Checkups:** Follow up with your orthodontist as recommended for retainer adjustments and progress checks.

- **Retainer Care:** If you have removable retainers, clean them daily with a soft toothbrush and mild soap or retainer cleaning tablets. Store them in their case when not in use.

- **Maintain Excellent Oral Hygiene:** Brush your teeth at least twice a day and floss daily. Pay extra attention to cleaning around your retainers or any bonded retainers.

- **Dietary Habits:** Continue to follow dietary guidelines that promote healthy teeth and avoid foods that could damage your retainers or teeth.

- **Protect Your Smile:** If you participate in contact sports, consider wearing a mouthguard to protect your teeth and orthodontic appliances.

- **Address Issues Promptly:** If you experience any issues, such as a loose retainer or discomfort, contact your orthodontist for guidance.

- **Maintain a Balanced Diet:** Stick to a balanced diet that supports overall health and oral health.

- **Avoid Harmful Habits:** Avoid habits like nail-biting, pen-chewing, or using your teeth as tools to prevent damage to your teeth and retainers.

9.3 Long-term Orthodontic Health

Long-term orthodontic health involves:

- **Commitment:** Be committed to wearing your retainers as instructed by your orthodontist. Consistency is key to maintaining your smile's alignment.

- **Communication:** If you experience any issues, questions, or concerns related to your orthodontic treatment, don't hesitate to reach out to your orthodontist for guidance and support.

- **Lifestyle Choices:** Make choices that support your oral health, including a balanced diet, regular exercise, and avoiding tobacco and excessive alcohol consumption.

- **Regular Dental Checkups:** Continue to schedule regular dental checkups to ensure your overall oral health is well-maintained.

- **Oral Hygiene:** Maintain excellent oral hygiene practices, including daily brushing, flossing, and using mouthwash as recommended.

- **Healthy Habits:** Avoid habits that could potentially harm your teeth, retainers, or overall health.

- **Patient Education:** Stay informed about oral health and orthodontic topics to make informed decisions about your care.

Long-term orthodontic health involves a commitment to your treatment plan, ongoing communication with your orthodontist, and a focus on maintaining overall oral health. By following these guidelines, you can enjoy the benefits of your orthodontic

treatment for years to come, including
a beautiful and healthy smile.